# The Let Them Theory Workbook: A Life-Changing Guide for Personal Transformation

(A Practical Workbook & Implementation Guide Inspired by Mel Robbins)

**SEAN ROBBINS**

**ISBN:** 978-1-300-46171-5

**Author:** Sean Robbins

**Book Title:** The Let Them Theory Workbook: A Life-Changing Guide for Personal Transformation (A Practical Workbook & Implementation Guide Inspired by Mel Robbins)

## SUMMARY

**The Let Them Theory: A Life-Changing Tool That Millios of People Can't Stop Talking About** (2024) is a transformative self-development book by Mel Robbins, a renowned motivational speaker, former CNN legal analyst, and bestselling author of *The 5 Second Rule* and *The High 5 Habit.*

Written at a time when interest in mental well-being and personal empowerment is at an all-time high, this book tackles a common issue—how people unknowingly give away their personal power by trying to control others or external situations. Drawing from her deep well of experience and insights from a social media following that has generated over 2 billion views, Robbins introduces a practical, actionable framework for reclaiming control over one's life.

At the heart of *The Let Them Theory* are two core principles:

- **"Let Them"**—a mindset shift that encourages readers to stop trying to control how others behave or respond.

- **"Let Me"**—a proactive approach that focuses on self-growth and personal agency through clear, actionable steps.

By blending psychology with real-world applications, Robbins walks readers through a structured path toward personal freedom. She explores key themes such as recognizing and reclaiming one's power, finding peace through non-attachment, and redirecting energy toward choices that truly empower.

This book isn't just about self-improvement—it's about unlocking a new way of living, one where you stop wasting energy on what you can't control and start focusing on what truly matters: your own growth and happiness.

This study guide refers to the 2024 Hay House e- book edition. Summary

**The Let Them Theory: A Revolutionary Approach to Personal Freedom and Growth**

Mel Robbins' *The Let Them Theory* (2024) introduces a powerful mindset shift that is reshaping the way people navigate relationships, personal growth, and emotional well-being. Drawing from her own experiences of struggle and transformation, Robbins presents a practical framework that empowers individuals to reclaim their personal agency, let go of unnecessary stress, and redirect their energy toward choices that truly matter.

At its core, *The Let Them Theory* is built on two key principles:

- **"Let Them"**—the practice of releasing the need to control how others think, act, or respond, creating space for peace and personal freedom.

- **"Let Me"**—a proactive shift toward self-empowerment, focusing on one's own growth rather than exhausting energy on external factors.

This concept first took shape when Robbins, caught up in trying to micromanage her son's high school prom, had an eye-opening realization: by simply letting go, she could free both herself and others from unnecessary tension. This insight, which she later shared in a viral social media video, ignited a global conversation about the liberating power of detachment and self-focus.

Through a blend of psychological insights, real-world applications, and personal anecdotes, Robbins explores how *The Let Them Theory* applies to different areas of life, including:


✓ **Managing Stress & Emotional Resilience** – Understanding what's within your control and shifting focus accordingly, supported by research from Harvard Medical School on stress reduction.

✓ **Family Dynamics** – Using the *Frame of Reference* tool to navigate complex relationships while maintaining emotional boundaries.

✓ **Friendships & Social Connections** – Embracing "The Great Scattering," the natural evolution of friendships, and understanding the Three Pillars of Friendship: proximity, timing, and energy.

✓ **Helping Others Without Enabling** – Applying the *ABC Loop* method (Apologize & Ask, Back off, Celebrate progress) to encourage accountability rather than rescuing people from their own growth.

✓ **Romantic Relationships** – Recognizing that actions, not words, reveal true feelings and that embracing non-attachment leads to healthier, more fulfilling connections.

Throughout the book, Robbins emphasizes that *The Let Them Theory* isn't about avoiding difficult conversations or tolerating harmful behavior—it's about making intentional choices that foster meaningful relationships and personal well-being. She likens life's challenges to weather patterns: while you can't control external circumstances, you *can* choose how you respond.

By integrating the principles of recognizing and reclaiming personal agency, embracing freedom through non-attachment, and redirecting energy toward empowering choices, *The Let Them Theory* provides a transformative roadmap for living with clarity, confidence, and peace.

The **Let Them Theory** builds on timeless philosophical ideas while applying them to modern-day personal growth and relationships. It merges wisdom from both Eastern and Western traditions, offering a fresh approach to self-empowerment, emotional independence, and maintaining healthy boundaries.

At its core, the theory reflects **Stoic philosophy**, particularly the distinction between what we can and cannot control. Like the Stoic thinker **Epictetus**, who believed freedom comes from accepting what's beyond our power, this framework encourages letting go of the need to control others' choices and emotions. The concept of **prohairesis**—the ability to make rational decisions regardless of external circumstances—closely aligns with Robbins's emphasis on emotional detachment and personal responsibility.

**Buddhist philosophy** also plays a role, especially in its principles of **non-attachment** as a path to reducing suffering. While traditional Buddhist teachings focus on releasing attachment to all desires, **The Let Them Theory** adapts this concept specifically to human relationships. Instead of trying to force situations to unfold a certain way, Robbins encourages embracing reality as it is. However, unlike Buddhism's focus on dissolving the ego, her approach prioritizes **personal empowerment and self-growth**.

The theory also echoes **existentialist** ideas, particularly **Jean-Paul Sartre's** concept of **radical responsibility**—the belief that individuals must take full ownership of their responses to life's circumstances. The "**Let Me**" component of Robbins's framework reflects this by emphasizing **proactive self-improvement**, rather than waiting for external validation or permission to change.

From a **psychological perspective**, the theory aligns with **Carl Jung's** ideas on **individuation**, which describe the lifelong process of developing a unique, authentic self while maintaining meaningful connections with others. Robbins's approach to **setting boundaries without sacrificing connection** mirrors this balance—encouraging personal growth without complete detachment from relationships.

Another key influence is **American Pragmatism**, particularly **William James's** idea that truth is determined by what "works" in real life. Robbins doesn't present her method as an **absolute** truth but as a **practical** tool that helps people navigate relationships, stress, and personal challenges effectively. The flexibility of the **Let Them Theory** allows individuals to adapt its principles to different situations, rather than following rigid rules.

The framework also draws from **contemporary feminist philosophy**, particularly its exploration of **autonomy within relationships**. Traditional Western philosophy often treats independence and relationships as opposing forces, but thinkers like **Carol Gilligan** argue that autonomy is not about isolation—it thrives within healthy relationships. Similarly, **The Let Them Theory** advocates for psychological independence while maintaining strong personal connections.

Beyond individual growth, the theory tackles **larger philosophical questions** about freedom and responsibility in an interconnected world. Unlike classical **individualism**, which views people as completely separate from one another, Robbins's perspective acknowledges deep human **interconnection** while still promoting **emotional independence**.

The book also introduces **epistemological themes**, particularly in its **Frame of Reference tool**, which helps people understand others' viewpoints without necessarily agreeing with them. This reflects **philosophical debates** on **relativism**—balancing the idea that multiple perspectives exist while still holding firm to one's own truth.

Finally, the theory ties into **virtue ethics**, focusing on **character development** rather than strict moral rules. Instead of prescribing universal guidelines, Robbins emphasizes the importance of cultivating traits like **emotional intelligence, self-awareness, and resilience**—an approach that mirrors **Aristotle's** belief that virtues develop through practice and habit.

In essence, **The Let Them Theory** is a **modern synthesis** of these philosophical traditions, designed for today's complex social and personal challenges. By blending **Eastern non-attachment, Western personal agency, feminist perspectives on autonomy, and pragmatic problem-solving**, it provides a structured yet adaptable path to personal growth, stronger relationships, and emotional freedom.

### INTRODUCTION SUMMARY: BREAKING FREE FROM CONTROL "MY STORY"

In *The Let Them Theory*, the author introduces a transformative approach to personal growth by shifting focus from controlling others to reclaiming individual power. The chapter opens with a deeply personal story of struggle—facing financial ruin, unemployment, and the collapse of her husband's business at 41. During this time, avoidance became a coping mechanism, leading to habits like oversleeping, drinking, and chronic procrastination.

Determined to change, she developed the *5 Second Rule*—a simple countdown method to override hesitation. After a TEDx talk propelled her into the spotlight, she became a sought-after motivational speaker. However, she soon realized that forcing action wasn't the real challenge—people constantly drained themselves trying to control others' reactions, emotions, and perceptions.

The breakthrough came with a simple yet powerful realization: *Let Them*. Instead of wasting energy managing how others perceive or respond, individuals can free themselves by letting go. This shift not only reduces stress but also strengthens relationships by fostering authentic connections. The chapter sets the stage for the book's core message—teaching readers how to redirect energy away from external validation and toward personal goals, growth, and self-fulfillment.

## PART 1, CHAPTER 1 SUMMARY: "STOP WASTING YOUR LIFE ON THINGS YOU CAN'T CONTROL"

In this chapter, Robbins shares how the *Let Them Theory* emerged from a pivotal moment involving her son, Oakley. When Oakley unexpectedly decided to attend prom at the last minute, Robbins became overwhelmed by the need to control the details — from dinner plans to a corsage she had bought for his date. The situation escalated when Robbins learned that Oakley and his friends had arranged a casual dinner, leading her and other parents to step in and try to manage things. However, her daughter Kendall stepped in, helping Robbins realize she needed to let go and allow her son to take charge of his evening.

This moment sparked Robbins' understanding of the importance of letting others make their own decisions and handle their own experiences — a concept that would later form the foundation of *The Let Them Theory*. As Robbins applied this principle to different areas of her life, including family dynamics and work-related situations, she noticed a significant decrease in stress and an increase in personal satisfaction. By refraining from trying to control other people's actions or reactions, Robbins discovered that she could focus her energy on what truly mattered: her own responses and growth.

The core message of the chapter is simple but powerful: While people may want to control external situations, the only real control they have lies in their own responses to those situations. This realization, Robbins suggests, can transform relationships and lead to a healthier emotional state.

### KEY TAKEAWAYS:

1. **Let Go of What You Can't Control**: Trying to control others' actions or decisions leads to frustration and stress. The only control you truly have is over your own response to situations.

2. **Emotional Detachment**: Learning to detach from the need to influence others' decisions can create peace and reduce anxiety.

3. **Personal Empowerment**: Focusing on how you react, rather than controlling others, fosters emotional growth and resilience.

4. **Relationships Improve**: Allowing others the freedom to handle their own lives enhances relationships by eliminating the tension of control.

- **Stress Reduction**: By releasing control, Robbins found relief from unnecessary stress.

- **Increased Satisfaction**: Not trying to control others' actions allowed Robbins to feel more fulfilled and peaceful.

## THE LIMITLESS POTENTIAL PLATEAU:

- By applying the *Let Them* principle consistently, Robbins discovered that she could break free from the exhausting cycle of managing others' expectations and reactions. This shift opened up limitless potential for personal growth.

**Results:**

- **Greater Peace**: The more Robbins practiced letting others make their own decisions, the more inner peace she gained.

- **Healthier Relationships**: By focusing only on her own actions and reactions, Robbins saw improvements in her family dynamics and work relationships.

## OBJECTIVES:

- **Release the Need to Control**: Practice letting go of the urge to control others' decisions.

- **Focus on Personal Responses**: Shift attention to how you respond to situations and people rather than trying to manage their behavior.

## METHODOLOGIES:

1. **Practice Emotional Detachment**: Recognize when you're trying to control a situation or person and actively choose to detach emotionally.

2. **Shift Focus to Your Own Growth**: Instead of worrying about others, focus on your own reactions and progress.

3. **Let Others Handle Their Own Experiences**: Allow friends, family, and coworkers to manage their choices without intervention.

1. **Identify Control Triggers**: Reflect on situations where you feel the need to control others. Write them down.

2. **Practice Letting Go**: The next time a similar situation arises, consciously step back and allow others to make their own decisions.

3. **Focus on Your Response**: Instead of reacting negatively, focus on how you can respond calmly and with understanding.

4. **Celebrate Progress**: Notice the changes in your stress levels and relationships as you practice letting go.

## *ACTION CHECKLIST:*

- ☐ Recognize when you're trying to control others.

- ☐ Take a step back and let them make their own choices.

- ☐ Redirect your focus to how you respond.

- ☐ Track your emotional growth and reduce stress over time.

By following this approach, you'll start breaking free from the constant need to control and begin focusing on what truly matters — your own peace and personal growth.

## PART 1, CHAPTER 2 SUMMARY: "GETTING STARTED: LET THEM + LET ME"

In this chapter, Robbins dives deeper into the two core concepts of *The Let Them Theory*: "Let Them" and "Let Me." She starts by sharing a personal experience where she found out, via social media, that several close friends had gone on a weekend trip without inviting her. This discovery triggered feelings of rejection and insecurity, sparking an emotional spiral where she questioned her worth and the strength of her friendships.

This experience serves as the foundation for the first component of the theory: "Let Them." Robbins explains that saying "Let Them" is a tool for emotional detachment, allowing you to accept others' actions without letting them dictate your emotional state. In her case, this meant accepting that her friends made their own choices, even though it initially felt painful. However, Robbins cautions that detachment, while providing temporary relief, can create a false sense of superiority and doesn't lead to true personal growth.

The second component of the theory, "Let Me," moves beyond passive acceptance into active self-empowerment. Robbins demonstrates how, after feeling left out, she examined her own role in maintaining friendships and focused on taking responsibility for her own choices. This shift allowed her to feel more in control of her own happiness without relying on others' actions.

As Robbins applies these principles across various aspects of her life — from family to work — she notices a dramatic reduction in stress and an increase in satisfaction. Her insights gained traction, especially after she shared them in a viral social media video, leading to a global conversation.

The core message of this chapter is that while we all have an innate desire to control our environments and relationships, the only true control we have is over our own reactions and responses to situations. By embracing both "Let Them" and "Let Me," Robbins positions this shift as essential for transforming personal relationships and emotional well-being.

### KEY TAKEAWAYS:

1. **Emotional Detachment ("Let Them")**: Learning to detach emotionally from others' choices helps maintain your peace and avoid unnecessary stress.

2. **Self-Empowerment ("Let Me")**: Taking responsibility for your own reactions and decisions leads to empowerment and personal growth.

3. **Control What You Can**: Recognize that the only thing you truly control is your response, not others' actions.

4. **Growth Comes from Within**: True emotional growth doesn't come from changing others, but from changing how you respond to them.

## MARGINAL GAINS:

- **Increased Self-Awareness**: By examining her own role in situations, Robbins became more aware of where she could improve and take control of her happiness.

- **Reduced Stress**: By letting go of the need to control others, Robbins noticed less emotional turbulence.

### THE LIMITLESS POTENTIAL PLATEAU:

- The concept of "Let Them + Let Me" provides a framework for breaking free from the limiting belief that you must control external factors to be happy. This realization unlocks limitless potential for personal growth.

**Results:**

- **Empowered Relationships**: By focusing on her own actions rather than trying to control others, Robbins experienced stronger, more authentic relationships.

- **Emotional Wellbeing**: Letting go of the need to manage others' reactions led to a greater sense of inner peace and satisfaction.

### OBJECTIVES:

- **Practice Emotional Detachment**: Let go of the need to control others' choices and focus on how you respond to them.

- **Own Your Reactions**: Shift from reacting passively to taking active responsibility for your emotional state.

### METHODOLOGIES:

1. **Apply "Let Them" in Real Life**: Practice letting go of the urge to influence or control others' decisions.

2. **Implement "Let Me" for Self-Examination**: Actively look at how your reactions shape your experiences and take ownership of your emotional responses.

3.  **Shift Focus to Your Own Growth**: Focus on your personal growth rather than trying to change others.

---

*ACTION PLAN:*

1.  **Identify Control Triggers**: Write down situations where you feel the urge to control others, like a disagreement or social exclusion.

2.  **Practice Letting Go**: The next time you face one of these triggers, practice stepping back and letting the situation unfold without intervention.

3.  **Examine Your Own Role**: After each situation, reflect on how your reactions impacted your emotional state and identify areas for improvement.

4.  **Shift Focus to Empowerment**: Rather than focusing on what others are doing, prioritize your own responses and growth.

## ACTION CHECKLIST:

- ☐ Recognize when you're trying to control others' actions.

- ☐ Practice letting them make their own choices.

- ☐ Take responsibility for how you respond emotionally.

- ☐ Reflect on your personal growth and track your emotional well-being.

By applying these steps, you'll begin to shift your mindset toward emotional independence, reducing stress, and fostering healthier, more fulfilling relationships.

In this chapter, Robbins addresses the universal challenge of managing stress in everyday life, especially when external factors, like others' actions or inconvenient situations, disrupt our emotional equilibrium. She highlights how small irritations—like technology failures or inconsiderate behavior—can build up over time, negatively affecting one's quality of life. Robbins argues that when we allow external events to dictate our emotional state, we lose our power and drain our energy unnecessarily.

To make her point, Robbins shares two personal stories. The first involves waiting in a long checkout line. Instead of giving in to frustration, Robbins uses the "Let Them" approach, reminding herself that the situation was beyond her control. In the second story, Robbins describes encountering a persistent coughing passenger on an airplane. Initially annoyed, she realized that she couldn't control the other person's behavior, but she could manage her own reaction.

Robbins then introduces expert insights from Dr. Aditi Nerurukar, a Harvard Medical School physician. Dr. Nerurukar explains that stress triggers a shift in brain function, moving from the prefrontal cortex (the logical, decision-making part) to the amygdala (responsible for survival responses). Over time, this shift can become chronic, with research showing that 70% of people live in a constant state of stress.

Robbins offers a two-step solution to managing stress using the "Let Them" theory. The first step involves recognizing what is out of our control by mentally saying, "Let Them." The second step empowers us to take control of our emotional responses with the phrase "Let Me" and by consciously breathing. Dr. Nerurukar supports this by explaining that deep breathing activates the vagus nerve, which helps restore normal brain function and reduces stress.

### KEY TAKEAWAYS:

1. **Small Irritations Add Up**: Everyday stressors, like waiting in line or dealing with rude behavior, can accumulate and drain our energy.

2. **Letting Go of Control**: The first step in managing stress is recognizing what is beyond your control and releasing the need to control it.

3. **Reclaim Your Power**: Focus on your emotional response rather than external circumstances.

4. **The Neuroscience of Stress**: Chronic stress impacts brain function, shifting focus away from logical thinking and decision-making.

5. **Breathe and Reset**: Conscious breathing can help reduce stress by activating the vagus nerve, restoring balance to the brain.

## MARGINAL GAINS:

- **Increased Emotional Awareness**: Recognizing when external factors trigger stress helps you regain control.

- **Stress Reduction**: By shifting focus from what you can't control to what you can, you experience less anxiety and more peace.

---

### THE LIMITLESS POTENTIAL PLATEAU:

- By mastering the art of letting go, you can break free from the limits imposed by stress. This awareness and control create an opening for unlimited personal growth.

**Results:**

- **Emotional Resilience**: Developing the ability to detach from stressful situations leads to more consistent emotional stability.

- **Improved Decision-Making**: When stress doesn't hijack your brain, you can think more clearly and make better decisions.

---

### OBJECTIVES:

- **Recognize Stress Triggers**: Identify situations that tend to stress you out and practice using the "Let Them" approach.

- **Regain Control**: Practice using "Let Me" to take charge of your emotional response to challenging situations.

---

### METHODOLOGIES:

1. **Acknowledge What You Can't Control**: The first step in managing stress is mentally acknowledging the situation is beyond your control.

2. **Focus on Your Response**: Shift your focus to how you can respond rather than trying to change the situation.

3. **Practice Conscious Breathing**: Incorporate deep breathing exercises to calm the nervous system and return to a balanced state.

---

*ACTION PLAN:*

1. **Identify Stress Points**: Write down moments throughout your day when you feel stressed or frustrated by external factors.

2. **Apply "Let Them"**: In each stressful situation, practice saying to yourself, "Let Them" to remind yourself of what you can't control.

3. **Take Control with "Let Me"**: After acknowledging the situation, use the "Let Me" approach to focus on your emotional response. Take a few deep breaths to regain your calm.

4. **Practice Daily**: Make these two steps part of your daily routine to manage stress more effectively.

## ACTION CHECKLIST:

- ☐ Recognize when you're giving too much emotional energy to things beyond your control.

- ☐ Practice saying "Let Them" to release the need to control external factors.

- ☐ Use "Let Me" to refocus on how you can manage your own reactions.

- ☐ Implement deep breathing techniques to calm your mind and restore balance.

By applying these steps consistently, you can reduce the stress in your life and increase your ability to respond to challenges with calm and clarity.

# PART 2, CHAPTER 4 SUMMARY: "LET THEM STRESS YOU OUT"

In Chapter 4, Robbins delves into how the "Let Them" approach can be used to manage stress in the workplace and other stressful situations. She starts by highlighting how workplace stress, particularly around career advancement, is a major source of stress for many people.

Robbins uses the example of an employee who, despite performing excellently, is denied a promotion. She encourages readers to shift their focus away from what they cannot control (like the unfairness of the situation) and instead focus on finding actionable solutions. She makes it clear that, while workplace situations may not always be fair, an individual's career progression is ultimately their responsibility—not their supervisor's.

Expanding the application of her theory, Robbins shares a personal story of a run-in with an irresponsible dog owner at a state park. This example illustrates that there's no one-size-fits-all response to stress. Sometimes confrontation is necessary, while other times reporting the incident or walking away is more appropriate. The flexibility of choosing your response based on the situation, your values, and your energy level is a key strength of the "Let Them" approach.

The chapter wraps up by applying this framework to the stress of political engagement. Robbins acknowledges how political polarization can be emotionally draining but urges readers to focus on what they can control—taking action where possible—rather than getting overwhelmed by external forces. She reinforces that while our initial stress reactions may be automatic, we have control over how we respond moving forward. The core message of this chapter is to channel energy away from things you can't control and into meaningful actions, reclaiming personal power and using the "Let Them" approach to reduce stress.

## KEY TAKEAWAYS:

- **Let Them**: Focus on what's within your control and stop stressing over uncontrollable situations.

- **Flexibility**: Adapt your response to each situation based on your values and energy levels.

- **Actionable Solutions**: Move from frustration to practical steps for improvement.

- **Control Your Response**: While initial reactions may be automatic, how you respond is always within your control.

## RELATED PROBLEMS:

- Workplace stress, particularly around career progression.

- Stress from unfair situations, such as being passed over for promotion or dealing with irresponsible people.

- Political stress and emotional overwhelm due to polarization.

## OBJECTIVES:

- Learn to distinguish between what you can and cannot control.

- Shift from frustration to proactive solutions.

- Practice responding to stressful situations with flexibility and focus on what you can change.

### ACTION PLAN:

1. **Identify Uncontrollable Stressors**: Recognize situations you cannot control.

2. **Shift Focus**: Redirect your energy towards what you can influence.

3. **Take Action**: Focus on actionable steps—whether it's having a conversation, seeking help, or walking away.

4. **Practice Emotional Detachment**: Use the "Let Them" method to detach from unnecessary emotional involvement in situations beyond your control.

## ACTION CHECKLIST:

- ☐ Identify a stressful situation you're currently facing.

- ☐ Ask yourself, "What part of this situation can I control?"

- ☐ Focus on what you can do and take one small step towards addressing it.

- ☐ Practice detaching emotionally from parts of the situation you can't control.

In *The Let Them Theory*, Mel Robbins introduces a transformative framework aimed at personal growth by teaching the art of letting go of control over external factors. This approach unfolds through a combination of relatable personal stories and scientific research, seamlessly integrating experiential and academic perspectives. Robbins begins by sharing a pivotal moment during her son's prom preparations, specifically the challenge she faced in letting go of control over dinner plans and the corsage situation. She reflects, "Little did I know that one moment would fundamentally change my entire approach to life" (25), marking the beginning of a profound shift in her mindset. This foundational story becomes the cornerstone of the broader practical and philosophical applications that follow.

The narrative structure moves from personal anecdotes to scientific evidence, such as the introduction of Dr. Aditi's neurological explanations on stress responses, bridging the gap between Robbins's lived experiences and empirical research. This progression not only makes the theory accessible but also credible, as Robbins provides both relatable examples and scientific backing. The chapter expands to demonstrate how the *Let Them* principle applies to various real-life situations, from navigating workplace dynamics to managing political stress, showcasing the theory's versatility.

A central theme of the book is **Recognizing and Reclaiming Personal Agency**. Robbins builds on this through Dr. Aditi's explanation of how stress affects the brain. Dr. Aditi highlights that "seven out of ten people are currently living in a chronic state of stress" (61), revealing how chronic stress can override rational decision-making and hinder personal growth. The theory provides a method for intervening in this automatic stress response by consciously choosing one's reactions, thereby regaining control over personal emotions and behaviors. This concept becomes crucial in environments like the workplace, where stress impacts decision-making and can limit career advancement.

Another key theme is **Freedom Through Non-Attachment**, which Robbins connects to Stoic and Buddhist teachings. She draws parallels between these ancient philosophies and modern psychological principles, illustrating how letting go of attachment to external circumstances fosters inner peace. Robbins ties this concept to *The Let Them Theory*, aligning it with Stoic beliefs that focus only on what can be controlled. For instance, the story of her son's prom serves as an example of relinquishing control for personal growth. Robbins contrasts passive acceptance with non-attachment, as seen in her response to feeling excluded by friends on a weekend trip. Instead of resigning to disappointment, she embraced non-attachment, which led to deeper personal growth.

In **Redirecting One's Energy Toward Empowering Choices**, Robbins encourages readers to rechannel their energy from stress and frustration into productive actions. She underscores the importance of this redirection in various contexts, such as seeking better job opportunities instead of staying in unfulfilling positions. Robbins offers numerous real-life scenarios where this redirection plays a crucial role, such as dealing with inconsiderate behavior in public or navigating difficult social interactions. By presenting a series of challenging situations and demonstrating how to redirect emotional energy toward positive outcomes, Robbins provides a clear, actionable methodology for applying the theory in daily life.

The analytical framework of *The Let Them Theory* blends multiple disciplines, integrating psychological research, neuroscience, ancient philosophy, and contemporary self-help methodologies. By referencing Dr. Aditi's work from Harvard Medical School on stress responses, Stoic philosophy through Epictetus, and Buddhist principles of non-attachment, Robbins strengthens her argument with evidence from diverse fields. This interdisciplinary approach supports the theory's core message: the importance of focusing on what can be controlled. The integration of Dr. Aditi's research on the brain's stress response mechanism alongside ancient wisdom effectively validates the concepts presented in the book, making it a holistic guide for personal transformation.

## KEY TAKEAWAYS:

- **Personal Agency**: You control your reactions, not the external stressors.
- **Non-Attachment**: Let go of what you cannot control to achieve inner peace.
- **Energy Redirection**: Shift your emotional energy from stress to proactive action.
- **Interdisciplinary Insights**: Combining neuroscience, philosophy, and psychology creates a well-rounded framework for growth.

## RELATED PROBLEMS:

- Chronic stress in personal and professional life.
- The challenge of letting go of control, especially in relationships or work situations.
- Difficulty in managing emotional responses to external circumstances.

## OBJECTIVES:

- Cultivate awareness of what you can and cannot control.
- Practice detachment from external circumstances to find peace.

- Redirect energy toward productive actions and solutions.

ACTION PLAN:

1. **Identify Stressors**: Recognize situations where you feel out of control and stressed.

2. **Shift Focus**: Concentrate on how you can respond, not what you can't control.

3. **Apply Non-Attachment**: Practice letting go of emotional attachment to outcomes.

4. **Redirect Energy**: Focus your emotional energy on actions that align with your values and goals.

## ACTION CHECKLIST:

- ☐ Acknowledge a stressful situation you cannot control.

- ☐ Practice detachment from external pressures and focus on your reaction.

- ☐ Choose one action that will shift your energy toward a solution.

- ☐ Reflect on how the redirection of energy improves your stress levels.

In Chapter 5 of *The Let Them Theory*, Mel Robbins tackles the pervasive fear of others' judgments and provides a method for overcoming it. She begins with a thought-provoking Mary Oliver quote: *"Tell me, what is it you plan to do with your one wild and precious life?"* (79), setting the stage for a discussion on how others' opinions inevitably influence life choices. Robbins argues that letting this fear control behavior traps individuals in a self-imposed prison, limiting their potential and happiness.

Robbins shares her own experience from the early stages of her career as a motivational speaker. Despite professional advice to leverage social media for business growth, she spent two years avoiding posting about her work online due to her fear of being judged by friends and acquaintances. This hesitation continued even as her family faced severe financial strain, illustrating how fear of judgment can hold people back from seizing opportunities.

The solution Robbins offers is to adopt *The Let Them Theory*: instead of trying to prevent or control negative opinions, simply let others think what they will. She explains that humans generate around 70,000 thoughts each day, many of which are random and beyond their control (86). Robbins emphasizes that while people may have fleeting negative thoughts about one another, these do not necessarily affect relationships or the quality of interactions, as seen in her own family's dynamic.

Robbins concludes the chapter by showing how the *Let Them* approach can be applied to decision-making. She highlights the importance of making choices based on personal values, rather than worrying about how others will react. When individuals make decisions out of guilt or fear of judgment, they lose control and often place blame on others. However, when they choose actions aligned with their values, they maintain their autonomy and self-respect, regardless of what others think.

### KEY TAKEAWAYS:

- **Fear of Judgment**: Fearing others' opinions can limit personal growth and happiness.

- **Let Them Think**: Allow people to have their opinions without trying to control or change them.

- **Make Decisions Based on Values**: Align choices with your personal values rather than seeking approval or avoiding judgment.

## RELATED PROBLEMS:

- Procrastination due to fear of judgment or criticism.

- Difficulty in making decisions based on what others might think.

- Struggling with guilt or people-pleasing behaviors.

## OBJECTIVES:

- Let go of the need for approval from others.

- Make decisions based on personal values rather than fear of others' opinions.

- Stop worrying about what others think and focus on your goals and values.

### ACTION PLAN:

1. **Acknowledge Fear of Judgment**: Identify moments when fear of what others will think holds you back.

2. **Apply Let Them**: Give others the freedom to have their opinions without trying to control or change them.

3. **Make Value-Driven Decisions**: When faced with choices, prioritize your own values instead of fearing others' reactions.

4. **Take Action**: Act confidently in decisions that align with your values, regardless of what others may think.

## ACTION CHECKLIST:

- ☐ Recognize when you are making decisions based on others' opinions.

- ☐ Consciously choose to let others have their thoughts without controlling them.

- ☐ Reflect on decisions made from your values, not guilt.

- ☐ Review your progress after making a decision that aligns with your true self.

### OVERVIEW

This chapter explores how to apply *The Let Them Theory* to family relationships, where emotional ties often make change more complex. Unlike friendships or workplace interactions, family systems operate as interconnected networks—when one person changes, the entire dynamic shifts. Robbins breaks down how to handle resistance, manage emotional responses, and cultivate compassion in difficult relationships.

### KEY TAKEAWAYS

1. **Family Systems Are Interconnected**

   o   When one person changes, their actions ripple through the family, triggering reactions.

   o   Family members often resist change more than friends or colleagues because shifts disrupt long-established roles and expectations.

2. **The Power of Perspective**

   o   Robbins shares her personal experience with her mother's disapproval of her marriage.

   o   Initially, she felt hurt, but later, she used the *Frame of Reference* technique (inspired by Lisa Bilyeu) to understand that her mother's concerns stemmed from her own past experiences, not outright rejection.

   o   Recognizing this allowed Robbins to separate emotional reactions from reality, leading to a more empathetic response.

3. **Accepting Multiple Truths**

   o   Understanding someone's perspective doesn't mean agreeing with it—it simply means acknowledging their reality.

   o   This approach helps manage difficult family dynamics, particularly in blended families, where patience and understanding are essential.

4. **Transformation Starts with You**

   o   While you can't control how family members think or feel, you can choose your response.

- Shifting your approach—whether by setting boundaries, practicing patience, or leading with compassion—can reshape the relationship over time.

---

*COMMON CHALLENGES & HOW TO OVERCOME THEM*

| Challenge | Solution |
|---|---|
| Family members resisting your changes | Understand that their reactions stem from their own fears or experiences, not necessarily from disapproval. |
| Feeling hurt by criticism or disapproval | Use the *Frame of Reference* technique to gain perspective before reacting emotionally. |
| Blended family struggles | Give relationships time to evolve, communicate openly, and focus on building trust rather than forcing bonds. |

......................................................................................................................................

*ACTION PLAN: APPLYING THE LET THEM THEORY IN FAMILY RELATIONSHIPS*

1. **Identify the Core Issue** – Determine whether resistance comes from fear, grief, or past experiences.

2. **Practice Emotional Detachment** – Don't take family reactions personally; instead, recognize their viewpoint.

3. **Shift Your Perspective** – Ask yourself: *What might be influencing their response?*

4. **Set Clear Boundaries** – Stand firm in your choices without trying to change their opinions.

5. **Lead with Compassion** – Approach conversations with understanding rather than defensiveness.

## FINAL THOUGHT

You don't have to agree with or even like every opinion your family holds. However, by choosing how you respond, you reclaim control over your emotions and interactions. *The Let Them Theory* isn't about changing others—it's about creating peace for yourself.

# PART 2, CHAPTER 7: WHEN GROWN-UPS THROW TANTRUMS

## SHORT SUMMARY

This chapter explores emotional maturity and how to navigate relationships with emotionally underdeveloped adults. Robbins emphasizes that while emotions are intense at any age, individuals should not take responsibility for managing another adult's emotional reactions. Instead, she introduces *The Let Them Theory* as a way to establish healthy boundaries while allowing others to experience their emotions without interference. She distinguishes between children—who need guidance in regulating their emotions—and adults, who must take ownership of their feelings.

---

### MARGINAL GAINS: SMALL SHIFTS FOR BIG IMPACT

- Recognizing that emotional outbursts in adults often stem from a lack of self-regulation.

- Shifting the mindset from trying to "fix" others to focusing on personal boundaries.

- Understanding that emotions are temporary and typically pass within seconds.

---

### THE LIMITLESS POTENTIAL PLATEAU

By embracing emotional maturity, individuals can transform how they interact with difficult people, reducing stress and increasing their ability to respond thoughtfully rather than react impulsively. This shift allows for stronger relationships and greater personal peace.

## KEY TAKEAWAYS

1. **Emotional Intensity Is Natural** – Adults feel emotions just as strongly as children, but managing them is a personal responsibility.

2. **Suppressed Emotions Cause Problems** – Clinical psychologist Dr. Lisa Damour explains that suppressing emotions leads to more dysfunction than openly experiencing them.

3. **Boundaries Protect Energy** – Instead of taking on another person's stress, let them process their feelings while maintaining personal space.

4. **Emotions Are Temporary** – Strong feelings last about six seconds chemically, so reacting impulsively only prolongs discomfort.

- Feeling obligated to calm down or "fix" emotionally volatile adults.

- Struggling to maintain boundaries with family members, colleagues, or partners who frequently express frustration, anger, or anxiety.

- Reacting impulsively to emotionally charged situations rather than choosing a measured response.

*OBJECTIVES TO REACH*

✅ Develop emotional resilience by focusing on personal reactions rather than external chaos.

✅ Learn to set and maintain healthy boundaries without guilt.

✅ Shift from reacting to emotions in the moment to responding with thoughtfulness.

✅ Recognize when to step back and let others handle their own emotional experiences.

*ACTION PLAN*

1. **Pause Before Responding** – When faced with an emotional outburst, take a breath instead of reacting immediately.

2. **Practice Letting Go** – Remind yourself that another person's emotions are not your responsibility.

3. **Set Clear Boundaries** – Decide in advance how you will handle emotional outbursts (e.g., walking away, offering limited support).

4. **Acknowledge Feelings Without Absorbing Them** – Validate another person's emotions without taking them on as your own.

5. **Reframe Emotional Maturity as a Skill** – View emotional intelligence as a lifelong learning process rather than an inherent trait.

## ACTION CHECKLIST

✅ Recognize that emotions are personal and not yours to manage.

✅ Allow others to feel what they feel without interference.

✅ Set personal boundaries to protect your energy.

✅ Choose thoughtful responses instead of emotional reactions.

✅ Accept that emotional maturity takes time and practice.

By implementing *The Let Them Theory* in emotionally charged situations, individuals can reclaim their peace, avoid unnecessary stress, and foster healthier relationships with those around them.

# PART 2, CHAPTER 8: THE RIGHT DECISION OFTEN FEELS WRONG

## SHORT SUMMARY

This chapter explores the difficulty of making necessary but emotionally challenging decisions. Robbins illustrates this with the story of a groom who hesitates before his wedding, despite the time, money, and expectations involved. She argues that people often avoid tough decisions out of fear of how others will react. Instead, she introduces *The Let Them Theory* as a framework for handling these moments: allowing others to feel their emotions (*Let Them*) while staying true to personal values (*Let Me*). She reinforces that avoiding necessary decisions to protect others' feelings can lead to long-term dissatisfaction in relationships and careers.

---

### MARGINAL GAINS: SMALL SHIFTS FOR BIG IMPACT

- Recognizing that discomfort doesn't mean a decision is wrong—it often signals growth.

- Shifting from external validation to internal clarity when making life choices.

- Understanding that emotions, like ocean waves, rise and fall naturally.

---

### THE LIMITLESS POTENTIAL PLATEAU

By embracing the emotional discomfort of difficult decisions, individuals unlock greater personal freedom, allowing them to align with their values rather than external pressures. This shift leads to more fulfilling relationships, careers, and life experiences.

## KEY TAKEAWAYS

1. **Difficult Decisions Are Often the Right Ones** – Fear of others' reactions can keep people stuck in situations that no longer serve them.

2. **Emotions Are Temporary** – Like ocean waves, feelings of fear or guilt rise and fall; they do not last forever.

3. **Avoiding Conflict Creates Bigger Problems** – Suppressing personal needs to keep others comfortable often leads to resentment and regret.

4. **You Are Not Responsible for Managing Others' Reactions** – People must be allowed to feel disappointment or frustration without interference.

## RELATED PROBLEMS

- Struggling to make decisions due to fear of disappointing others.

- Staying in unfulfilling relationships, careers, or commitments to avoid conflict.

- Feeling overwhelmed by emotional reactions when making tough choices.

### OBJECTIVES TO REACH

✓ Develop the confidence to make decisions based on personal values, not external expectations.

✓ Accept emotional discomfort as part of growth rather than a sign of failure.

✓ Stop taking responsibility for managing others' emotional responses.

✓ Strengthen emotional independence by practicing *The Let Them Theory* in daily life.

### ACTION PLAN

1. **Recognize Fear as a Normal Part of Change** – Acknowledge that making a big decision will bring temporary discomfort.

2. **Detach from Others' Reactions** – Let people process their emotions without trying to fix or minimize their feelings.

3. **Use the Emotional Wave Metaphor** – When emotions feel overwhelming, remind yourself that they will pass.

4. **Prioritize Long-Term Well-Being Over Short-Term Comfort** – Stay focused on what aligns with your values rather than immediate approval.

5. **Reaffirm Personal Boundaries** – Make choices that serve your growth, even if they upset others.

## ACTION CHECKLIST

✓ Accept that hard decisions don't always feel good in the moment.

✓ Acknowledge that emotions, like waves, come and go.

✓ Stop delaying decisions out of fear of others' reactions.

✓ Practice emotional independence by focusing on what aligns with your future.

✓ Trust that choosing personal fulfillment will lead to long-term happiness.

By applying *The Let Them Theory*, individuals can navigate emotionally tough decisions with confidence, allowing themselves and others the space to grow and adapt.

# CHAPTER 9: LIFE ISN'T ALWAYS FAIR—BUT THAT'S OKAY

## SUMMARY

In this chapter, Robbins tackles a hard truth—life isn't fair. Instead of resisting this reality, she argues that accepting it frees individuals from the toxic cycle of comparison. The more people fixate on what others have, the less energy they have to focus on their own growth.

She introduces two types of comparison:

- **Upward Comparison** – Looking at those who seem more successful, privileged, or talented and feeling inadequate.

- **Downward Comparison** – Recognizing one's advantages by comparing them to those in less fortunate circumstances.

Robbins shares a personal story about her daughter Sawyer, who struggled with self-esteem by constantly comparing herself to her sister Kendall's different talents and physical attributes. She highlights how focusing on unchangeable traits—like family background, genetics, or physical characteristics—only drains energy that could be used to improve areas within one's control.

The chapter also addresses the mental health risks of excessive comparison. Studies show that an obsessive need to control unchangeable aspects of life can fuel anxiety, depression, and even self-destructive behaviors. Robbins emphasizes the importance of shifting perspective—choosing gratitude over resentment and focusing on personal growth rather than unfair circumstances.

---

*MARGINAL GAINS: SMALL SHIFTS THAT MAKE A BIG DIFFERENCE*

- Recognizing the difference between what you can and can't control

- Redirecting energy from comparison to personal improvement

- Practicing gratitude to counteract feelings of inadequacy

- Shifting from a competitive mindset to a growth-focused one

---

*THE LIMITLESS POTENTIAL PLATEAU*

By letting go of resentment over life's unfairness, individuals can unlock greater emotional freedom and confidence. Instead of feeling stuck in comparison, they begin seeing opportunities where they once saw obstacles.

## KEY TAKEAWAYS

- Life isn't fair, and focusing on that fact won't change anything.

- Comparison—especially to factors outside your control—prevents growth.

- True fulfillment comes from progress, not from measuring up to others.

- A mindset shift from competition to collaboration improves mental well-being.

## COMMON PROBLEMS RELATED TO THIS TOPIC

1. **Low Self-Esteem** – Constant comparison erodes self-worth.

2. **Anxiety & Depression** – A focus on life's unfairness fuels stress and unhappiness.

3. **Lack of Motivation** – When people feel they can't "win," they stop trying.

4. **Bitterness & Resentment** – Fixation on others' advantages leads to negativity.

### OBJECTIVES YOU WANT TO REACH

- Accept life's unfairness without letting it define you.

- Develop resilience by focusing on what *you* can improve.

- Stop self-sabotage by eliminating toxic comparison habits.

- Foster a mindset that values collaboration over competition.

### YOUR ACTION PLAN

✓ Identify areas where comparison is limiting your happiness.
✓ Write down things you *can* change and commit to improving them.
✓ Practice gratitude daily—list three things you're thankful for.
✓ Whenever you catch yourself comparing, reframe it as motivation.
✓ Surround yourself with people who encourage growth, not competition.

By embracing *The Let Them Theory*, Robbins encourages readers to let go of the frustration of life's inequalities and refocus on their personal journey. Instead of competing, they can channel their energy into becoming the best version of themselves.

# PART 2, CHAPTER 10: HOW TO MAKE COMPARISON YOUR TEACHER

## SUMMARY

In this chapter, Robbins redefines comparison—not as a destructive force but as a powerful teacher. Instead of allowing jealousy or self-doubt to take over, she encourages readers to shift their mindset: use comparison as fuel for improvement rather than a source of frustration.

She differentiates between **harmful comparison**, which leads to self-pity and resentment, and **productive comparison**, which highlights areas for growth and change. By focusing on what *can* be improved instead of dwelling on what's unchangeable, individuals can turn envy into action.

---

*MARGINAL GAINS: SMALL SHIFTS THAT MAKE A BIG DIFFERENCE*

- Instead of resenting others' success, use it as proof of what's possible.

- Recognize when comparison is pushing you toward self-sabotage.

- Shift from a mindset of competition to one of inspiration.

- Take personal responsibility for the outcomes you desire.

---

*THE LIMITLESS POTENTIAL PLATEAU*

When individuals stop seeing others' success as a threat and start viewing it as a roadmap, they unlock greater possibilities. Every achievement they envy can become a lesson in what is possible for them as well.

## KEY TAKEAWAYS

- Comparing yourself to others can either hold you back or push you forward.

- The difference lies in how you interpret the success of others.

- Rather than focusing on what you lack, study what they did to achieve success.

- "Let Them" succeed and "Let Me" take control of my own path.

## CASE STUDIES: REAL-LIFE TRANSFORMATIONS

### 1. Molly, the Interior Designer

Molly felt frustrated when an inexperienced competitor gained traction on social media. Instead of validating her frustration, Robbins challenged her to view this as an opportunity. The real issue wasn't the competitor's success—it was Molly's reluctance to adapt. Once she embraced online marketing, she transformed her business.

### 2. Robbins' Personal Money Mindset Shift

When Robbins visited a friend's beautifully renovated home while struggling with debt, she felt a deep sense of jealousy. But this moment led to an eye-opening realization—she had placed responsibility for financial success solely on her husband. Instead of staying stuck in resentment, she decided to take charge of her career, a shift that took 15 years of consistent effort but ultimately changed her life.

## COMMON PROBLEMS RELATED TO COMPARISON

1. **Self-Doubt** – Feeling like you're not good enough when others succeed.

2. **Stagnation** – Allowing envy to discourage action instead of inspiring it.

3. **Victim Mindset** – Believing success is unfairly distributed rather than earned.

4. **Lack of Accountability** – Failing to take responsibility for personal growth.

---

### OBJECTIVES YOU WANT TO REACH

- Shift from resenting others' success to learning from it.

- Identify opportunities for personal growth instead of feeling stuck.

- Replace competition with inspiration.

- Take full ownership of your progress and results.

### YOUR ACTION PLAN

✓ When you feel jealous, ask: *What does this person's success teach me?*

✓ Identify one thing you admire in someone else—then take one action to improve in that area.

✓ Replace negative self-talk with constructive questions: *What can I do differently?*

✓ Create a personal success plan instead of dwelling on what others have.

✓ Remind yourself: *Their success does not take away from mine.*

By embracing *The Let Them Theory*, Robbins encourages readers to stop seeing others' success as a threat and instead use it as a roadmap for their own growth. The key is shifting from competition to curiosity—learning, adapting, and taking responsibility for personal success.

## ANALYSIS OF PART 2, CHAPTERS 5-10

In Chapters 5-10 of *The Let Them Theory*, Robbins builds a compelling case for personal agency and emotional independence, carefully developing her argument through a series of interconnected chapters. Each chapter addresses different facets of letting go of external validation, moving from fear of others' opinions to managing emotional reactions and comparing oneself to others. Through a combination of personal anecdotes, psychological research, and practical advice, Robbins constructs a framework that encourages self-determination and emotional freedom. The chapters work together systematically to deepen readers' understanding of these concepts, using storytelling to introduce new ideas and expand them into actionable insights.

### KEY THEMES AND CONCEPTS

1. **Recognizing and Reclaiming Personal Agency**
   A dominant theme throughout these chapters is recognizing and reclaiming personal agency. Robbins argues that people lose their sense of agency when they focus on managing others' emotional responses or seeking external validation. This surrender of control manifests in various aspects of life, including career choices and personal relationships. *The Let Them Theory* becomes the tool for regaining this agency by acknowledging the limitations of controlling others and shifting that energy toward personal growth and decision-making.

2. **Freedom Through Non-Attachment**
   Robbins introduces the concept of emotional non-attachment as a powerful means of gaining emotional freedom. She breaks down emotions scientifically, explaining that they are brief chemical reactions that last only about six seconds. By understanding that emotions are temporary, Robbins advocates for embracing them without trying to suppress or control them. This shift away from emotional attachment reduces suffering and promotes a healthier, more balanced emotional state.

3. **Redirecting Energy Toward Empowering Choices**
   Robbins repeatedly encourages readers to focus their energy on making empowering choices. Instead of viewing emotions like jealousy as negative, she reframes them as opportunities for growth. She explains that jealousy can be seen as an invitation to envision a better future self by observing what others have accomplished. This perspective transforms potentially harmful emotions into catalysts for positive change and self-improvement. Robbins provides real-

life examples where this redirection has led to progress in personal and professional development.

4. **The Power of Metaphors**

   Robbins uses metaphors to help clarify complex ideas, with the *web metaphor* standing out as a key tool for understanding family dynamics. She describes family systems as interconnected webs, where a change made by one individual can send either positive or negative ripples through the entire system. This powerful imagery helps readers comprehend the intricacies of personal and familial change, showing how growth in one area can influence the whole.

5. **The Role of Psychological Research**

   Robbins strengthens her arguments with references to psychological research, incorporating expert opinions from professionals like Dr. Lisa Damour and Dr. Anne Davin. These references lend scientific credibility to Robbins's framework, particularly in her discussions of emotional responses and boundaries. The research on "upward comparison" (comparing oneself to those perceived as superior) and "downward comparison" (comparing oneself to those in less favorable circumstances) provides a nuanced understanding of the effects of comparison, further reinforcing her points about redirecting focus from others to oneself.

## BROADER IMPLICATIONS

The underlying message of these chapters is that personal growth comes from within and is not dependent on managing others' emotions or comparing yourself to them. Robbins encourages readers to embrace emotional independence, shifting from external validation to internal growth. The chapters also stress the importance of accepting emotions as natural and transient, rather than letting them control your actions or sense of self-worth. By taking responsibility for their own emotions and choices, individuals can live more authentic and fulfilling lives.

## ACTIONABLE TAKEAWAYS

- **Reclaim Your Agency**: Stop trying to control others' opinions or emotional reactions. Instead, focus on making decisions that align with your values and growth.

- **Embrace Emotional Non-Attachment**: Recognize that emotions are brief and temporary. Instead of suppressing or reacting impulsively, acknowledge them and allow yourself to move through them.

- **Reframe Jealousy and Comparison**: See jealousy as an opportunity for personal growth. Use others' success as motivation to reflect on your own potential and goals.

- **Use Metaphors to Understand Change**: Understand that changes in your life can have far-reaching effects, especially within your family dynamics. Embrace the interconnectedness of relationships and use this awareness to guide your personal transformation.

- **Implement The Let Them Theory**: Use this framework to create healthy boundaries, prioritize emotional independence, and empower your choices in relationships, work, and personal life.

Through these practical strategies, Robbins guides readers toward embracing their emotional independence and reclaiming control over their lives. By reframing negative emotions and letting go of comparison, individuals can unlock their potential for growth and fulfillment.

In Chapter 11, Robbins dives into the complexities of adult friendships, shedding light on a transition that many face after high school or college, which she terms "The Great Scattering." This phase marks the period when close-knit friend groups tend to disperse, often leaving individuals feeling disconnected or uncertain about maintaining friendships as adults. Robbins contrasts childhood friendships, which are often facilitated by structured environments like schools and extracurricular activities, with the challenges that come with sustaining meaningful connections in adulthood.

Robbins introduces the concept of the "Three Pillars of Friendship," which are *proximity*, *timing*, and *energy*. Each of these factors plays a crucial role in how friendships evolve over time:

- **Proximity**: The University of Kansas research shows that casual friendships require about 74 hours of interaction, and close friendships demand over 200 hours. The more time you spend with someone, the closer the relationship tends to become.

- **Timing**: Robbins explains that people in similar life stages naturally share more in common, which facilitates stronger connections. As life stages change, so too do the dynamics of relationships.

- **Energy**: This pillar refers to the intangible connection between individuals, which can fluctuate. It's the energy that fuels interactions, and it can change over time based on the life circumstances or priorities of the individuals involved.

The chapter emphasizes the importance of accepting the natural cycles of friendships rather than trying to force connections to persist. Robbins references the common saying that some friendships exist for a season, others for a specific reason, and a few endure for a lifetime. She illustrates this point with a personal story of being excluded from a friend group, which helped her understand the need to adapt to changing dynamics. Ultimately, Robbins encourages readers to let go of rigid expectations about friendships and adopt a more flexible, understanding view of adult relationships.

# PART 3, CHAPTER 12 SUMMARY: "WHY SOME FRIENDSHIPS NATURALLY FADE"

In Chapter 12, Robbins delves into the natural evolution of friendships, using her personal experiences to highlight how the three pillars of friendship—*proximity*, *timing*, and *energy*—influence the longevity and changes within relationships.

Robbins shares a story where a close friend of hers moved near two other couples in their social circle, leading to a shift in the dynamic. As these three families grew closer due to physical proximity, Robbins found herself feeling increasingly excluded. She acknowledges that her response was emotionally immature, experiencing jealousy and acting out negatively at social gatherings, while her husband handled the changes without taking them personally.

Through this example, Robbins illustrates how adult friendships often change due to shifts in *proximity*, *timing*, or *energy*. She reflects on her own life changes—such as relocating and running a growing business—that impacted her ability to stay in regular contact with friends. This example reinforces how life circumstances can naturally affect the closeness of relationships.

The chapter concludes with Robbins advocating for a more flexible, understanding approach to friendship. She encourages readers to maintain goodwill towards friends who may become distant and stay open to the possibility of reconnection. Robbins demonstrates this with her own experience of reconciling with the couples from her story, showing that relationships can endure even after periods of distance, as long as they are approached with maturity and openness.

## PART 3, CHAPTER 13 SUMMARY: "HOW TO CREATE THE BEST FRIENDSHIPS OF YOUR LIFE"

In Chapter 13, Robbins delves into the process of forming deep, meaningful friendships as an adult. Building on previous concepts like "The Great Scattering" and the three pillars of friendship (proximity, timing, and energy), Robbins presents these ideas as essential tools for understanding how adult relationships evolve.

She draws on her personal experience of moving to a small town at age 54. After a year of isolation, Robbins's daughters encouraged her to reach out to a neighbor, which marked the beginning of her journey to integrate into the community. This led her to develop a method called the "going first" strategy, where you take the initiative to introduce yourself, show interest in others, and make connections.

Robbins highlights the importance of "weak ties"—casual acquaintances that can eventually turn into significant friendships. She shares how she systematically built relationships with regular patrons and staff at a local coffee shop, using details about their lives to foster deeper connections over time.

She provides four core strategies for forming new friendships:

1.  Ask about others' experiences.

2.  Show genuine interest in their lives.

3.  Maintain an approachable demeanor.

4.  Avoid the expectation of instant friendship.

The chapter concludes with Robbins's belief that patience is key in building a social network. Drawing from her own experience and her daughter's college transition, Robbins encourages readers to give it time—"Give it a year"—as relationships require consistent effort and engagement to develop.

### IMPORTANT TAKEAWAYS:

1.  **Initiate Connections**: Taking the first step is essential. Don't wait for others to approach you—be the one to start the conversation and show interest.

2.  **"Weak Ties" Matter**: Casual acquaintances can evolve into meaningful friendships over time with effort and shared experiences.

3.  **Patience Pays Off**: Building strong friendships as an adult is a gradual process. Give relationships time to develop naturally.

4. **Four Key Strategies for Friendship**:

   o   Ask questions to learn more about others.

   o   Show genuine interest in their responses.

   o   Maintain an approachable and friendly demeanor.

   o   Don't rush—allow friendships to grow without expectation.

## RELATED PROBLEMS:

- **Difficulty in forming new friendships**: Many adults struggle with making new friends due to time constraints, geographic relocation, or fear of rejection.

- **Impatience in relationship-building**: People often expect quick results, leading to disappointment when relationships don't immediately flourish.

## OBJECTIVES TO REACH:

1. Develop a strategy for initiating meaningful friendships.

2. Shift perspective on casual acquaintances to recognize their potential for deeper connections.

3. Cultivate patience in the process of forming lasting relationships.

## YOUR ACTION PLAN:

1. **Take Initiative**: Identify potential connections in your community or workplace. Introduce yourself and start conversations.

2. **Use the "Going First" Strategy**: Be the one to make the first move. Show genuine interest in others by asking questions and engaging in active listening.

3. **Track Progress**: Keep track of your interactions, noting names, details, and interests of people you meet to build deeper connections over time.

4. **Be Patient**: Understand that friendships take time to form. Don't rush the process; instead, give relationships time to evolve naturally.

## ACTION CHECKLIST:

- ☐ Reach out to one person each week to initiate a new connection.

- ☐ Make note of details (names, hobbies, interests) to remember and personalize future interactions.

- ☐ Show up consistently in social environments where potential friendships can grow (e.g., coffee shops, local clubs).

- ☐ Allow at least six months to a year before evaluating the depth of a new friendship.

- ☐ Be patient and stay open to the natural rhythms of friendship development.

By following these steps, you'll actively cultivate new friendships and create a supportive social network that can enrich your life for years to come.

## PART 3, CHAPTER 14 SUMMARY: "PEOPLE ONLY CHANGE WHEN THEY FEEL LIKE IT"

In Chapter 14, Robbins explores the concept of motivation and why trying to change others often fails. She uses a case study about a woman attempting to improve her husband's health habits, illustrating how external pressure can create resistance and strain relationships, even when the intentions are good.

Robbins introduces three key principles about motivation:

1. **Adults only change when they are internally motivated.**

2. **External pressure cannot create authentic motivation.**

3. **People often believe they are exceptions to negative consequences.**

She backs these ideas with research from Dr. Tali Sharot, a behavioral neuroscientist, who discovered that the brain deactivates when receiving unwanted advice or warnings, which makes traditional methods of motivation ineffective.

The chapter goes on to examine how attempting to influence others' behavior often leads to power struggles. When someone feels pressured to change, they resist in order to preserve their autonomy, even if they want the change. This creates what Robbins calls a "gridlock" that grows over time.

To resolve this, Robbins advocates for **The Let Them Theory**—accepting others as they are and giving them the space to make changes at their own pace. She argues that when you stop applying pressure, you create an environment where genuine transformation can occur naturally.

### IMPORTANT TAKEAWAYS:

1. **Internal Motivation Is Key**: People are most likely to change when they feel internally driven, not when pressured by others.

2. **Pressure Leads to Resistance**: Attempting to change others through external influence often backfires, creating resistance and tension.

3. **People See Themselves as Exceptions**: Many individuals believe that negative consequences won't apply to them, which makes them less likely to listen to advice.

4. **The Let Them Theory**: The most effective way to encourage change is by allowing others to make their own decisions and change on their own terms.

## RELATED PROBLEMS:

- **Strained relationships**: Pressure to change others can lead to frustration and power struggles, often damaging relationships.

- **Ineffective motivation**: Well-intentioned advice or warnings can be met with resistance if it's perceived as an attempt to control.

## OBJECTIVES TO REACH:

1. Recognize that motivating others through pressure rarely works.

2. Learn to accept others as they are and trust them to make their own decisions.

3. Shift from trying to change others to focusing on encouraging natural growth and change at their own pace.

## YOUR ACTION PLAN:

1. **Let Go of Control**: Stop trying to force others to change. Focus on supporting their autonomy instead of pressuring them.

2. **Provide Encouragement, Not Advice**: Offer support and encouragement without trying to push others in a specific direction. Let them come to their own conclusions.

3. **Create Space for Change**: Give people the time and space to change on their own terms. Understand that change often happens when it feels natural, not when it's forced.

## ACTION CHECKLIST:

- ☐ Identify one relationship where you are trying to motivate someone to change. Reflect on how you can stop applying pressure and allow the person space for growth.

- ☐ Practice offering support rather than advice in your conversations. Focus on creating an environment where the other person feels heard and respected.

- ☐ Monitor your reactions when someone resists your suggestions. Take a step back and remind yourself that true change comes from within.

- ☐ Be patient and trust that others will change in their own time. Give them the freedom to make decisions without feeling like they are being pushed.

By following these strategies, you can foster healthier, more respectful relationships that allow for natural growth and transformation.

## PART 3, CHAPTER 15 SUMMARY: "UNLOCK THE POWER OF YOUR INFLUENCE"

In Chapter 15, Robbins explores a more effective way to influence behavioral change in others by focusing on acceptance and modeling desired behaviors rather than applying pressure. Drawing from research on human nature, Robbins explains that people tend to mimic behaviors they observe in others, especially when those behaviors seem enjoyable or beneficial.

Robbins introduces the **ABC Loop method** for facilitating change, which involves three key steps:

1.  **Apologize and Ask**: Begin with an open-ended, pressure-free discussion, asking questions and focusing on listening rather than offering advice.

2.  **Back Off**: After the initial conversation, step back and allow the person to make their own choices, recognizing that change may take time—sometimes up to six months or more.

3.  **Celebrate Progress**: Reinforce positive changes immediately by celebrating progress, no matter how small, to create a positive association with the new behavior.

Before applying the ABC Loop, Robbins recommends examining one's motivations for wanting others to change. Self-reflection helps identify any unconscious need for control and sets the stage for more effective and respectful conversations.

The chapter emphasizes that patience is key, as change doesn't always happen overnight, and the ABC Loop may need to be repeated. While this method can be powerful, Robbins acknowledges that it doesn't guarantee change in others, but it creates an environment where change is more likely to occur organically.

### IMPORTANT TAKEAWAYS:

1.  **Modeling Behavior**: Instead of applying pressure, model the behavior you want to see in others. People are more likely to adopt behaviors they observe, especially when those behaviors seem enjoyable or beneficial.

2.  **The ABC Loop**: A pressure-free, supportive approach to influencing change:

    o   **Apologize and Ask**: Start by listening, not advising.

- o **Back Off**: Give the person space to change on their own time.

- o **Celebrate Progress**: Reinforce positive behavior through celebration.

3. **Patience is Key**: Change takes time, and you might need to repeat the ABC Loop multiple times to see results. Give people the space to grow at their own pace.

4. **Self-Reflection**: Before trying to change others, examine your motivations. Understanding your desire for control helps you approach the situation more effectively and compassionately.

## RELATED PROBLEMS:

- **Impatience**: Expecting immediate results can lead to frustration and ineffective attempts to influence others.

- **Need for Control**: A strong desire to change others can be rooted in an unconscious need for control, which can sabotage efforts to build positive relationships.

- **Resistance to Change**: Even with the best intentions, trying to force change can cause resistance and strain relationships.

### OBJECTIVES TO REACH:
1. Learn to influence others by modeling the behaviors you want to see.

2. Use the ABC Loop to create a supportive environment for change without applying pressure.

3. Cultivate patience and allow others the time they need to make changes.

4. Reflect on your motivations for wanting others to change and ensure you're acting out of a desire for genuine improvement, not control.

### YOUR ACTION PLAN:
1. **Practice Active Listening**: In your conversations, focus more on listening than advising. Try to understand the other person's perspective and ask open-ended questions to encourage dialogue.

2. **Give Space for Growth**: After your initial discussion, step back and allow the person time to make their own decisions. Recognize that change doesn't happen instantly.

3. **Celebrate Progress**: Whenever you notice progress, even small steps, celebrate it. Positive reinforcement will help build an association between new behaviors and positive outcomes.

4. **Self-Reflect**: Before trying to influence someone, ask yourself why you want them to change. Make sure you're coming from a place of compassion and understanding rather than a need for control.

## ACTION CHECKLIST:

- ☐ Reflect on your motivations for wanting to influence someone's behavior. Are you trying to control the situation or genuinely support their growth?

- ☐ Practice the ABC Loop in your next interaction. Start by listening and asking open-ended questions, then step back and celebrate any positive changes.

- ☐ Be patient and understanding if the person doesn't change immediately. Remind yourself that real transformation takes time.

- ☐ Celebrate any progress, no matter how small, and reinforce the positive behaviors you want to see.

By following the ABC Loop and focusing on modeling behavior rather than applying pressure, you can create a more supportive and effective environment for change, helping others grow at their own pace.

In Chapters 11-15, Robbins lays out a comprehensive framework for understanding adult friendships and personal change, structured around three key pillars: **proximity, timing, and energy**. The author introduces the concept of **"The Great Scattering"**, describing how post-college life disrupts established social networks, forcing individuals to navigate and rebuild relationships on their own. Through personal anecdotes and detailed examples, Robbins explains how these shifting dynamics affect how we form and maintain friendships as adults. A significant empirical reference from the University of Kansas highlights the time investment needed to form meaningful friendships, with **74 hours** required to establish a casual bond (162). This data reinforces the complexity of adult friendship development and offers a scientific foundation for Robbins' exploration of relationship dynamics.

Robbins also touches on the theme of **Freedom Through Non-Attachment** when she discusses the necessity of letting go of rigid expectations in adult friendships. Drawing from personal experiences of evolving social circles, Robbins argues that attachment to specific outcomes in relationships only leads to disappointment and suffering. She states, **"The reality is, adult friendships come and go. Expecting friendship will destroy it"** (160). The text promotes flexibility, suggesting that we should accept the natural ebb and flow of relationships as part of life's broader transitions, ultimately finding freedom through non-attachment.

The theme of **Recognizing and Reclaiming Personal Agency** is evident throughout the chapters, particularly when Robbins discusses why efforts to motivate others to change typically fail. By referencing research from **Dr. Tali Sharot** and other behavioral neuroscientists, Robbins shows that attempts to pressure others into change are counterproductive. Instead, she advocates for **The Let Them Theory**, which emphasizes allowing others to make changes on their own terms, backed by neurological insights on decision-making. Robbins introduces the **ABC Loop Method** (Apologize, Back Off, Celebrate) as a structured approach to encourage personal change in others without encroaching on their autonomy.

Robbins further explores the concept of **Redirecting One's Energy Toward Empowering Choices** in her discussion of influence versus control. Using research on **social contagion** from Dr. Sharot, Robbins explains that behavior change is more effective when modeled rather than forced. She uses examples from various domains, including work and personal relationships, to show how positive behavior can inspire others to adopt similar practices. The text reinforces this idea by showcasing how redirecting energy from control to influence can produce more lasting and meaningful outcomes. Through motivational interviewing techniques, Robbins demonstrates that fostering a space for others to come to their own conclusions leads to better results.

The text employs several rhetorical devices, particularly **extended metaphors** and **parallel structures**, to strengthen its message. The recurring metaphor of "scattering"— to describe life transitions—creates a cohesive thread throughout the narrative. Robbins builds her credibility by seamlessly combining **personal anecdotes**, **scientific research**, and **practical strategies**. This combination of the theoretical with the real-world ensures the reader remains engaged while understanding complex psychological principles.

The chapters heavily rely on **psychological research** and **behavioral science** to support the central arguments about relationships and personal growth. Robbins references studies from institutions like the University of Kansas and University College London, weaving these findings into her narrative to demonstrate the practical applications of complex psychological concepts. Through her use of case studies and personal stories, Robbins makes her theoretical framework accessible and actionable, solidifying the book's focus on real-world implementation.

## KEY THEMES AND INSIGHTS:

1. **The Great Scattering & Friendship Dynamics**: The post-college phase challenges friendship formation, requiring adaptability and understanding of how **proximity**, **timing**, and **energy** affect relationships.

2. **Freedom Through Non-Attachment**: Letting go of rigid expectations in friendships leads to emotional freedom and acceptance of relationships as they evolve naturally over time.

3. **Personal Agency & Change**: True change in others only happens when they feel internally motivated, not under external pressure. The **ABC Loop** (Apologize, Back Off, Celebrate) offers a framework to encourage change without compromising autonomy.

4. **Redirecting Energy Toward Empowering Choices**: Influence, not control, is the most effective method for encouraging change. By modeling desired behaviors, you create a space for others to adopt them voluntarily, leading to positive outcomes.

5. **Psychological and Behavioral Science Integration**: The text uses research and case studies to validate the core principles of relationship management, behavioral change, and personal growth.

## PRACTICAL APPLICATION AND TAKEAWAYS:

1. **Friendship Development**: Understand that adult friendships require time and effort, with proximity, timing, and energy being key factors. Accept that some relationships are seasonal or temporary, and don't be afraid to let go of expectations.

2. **Non-Attachment in Relationships**: Avoid clinging to specific outcomes in your friendships and relationships. Embrace the natural ebb and flow of connections to minimize disappointment and cultivate peace.

3. **Support Others' Change**: Encourage change in others by adopting the **ABC Loop Method**: Start by listening and apologizing (when necessary), step back to give them room, and celebrate their progress along the way.

4. **Influence Over Control**: Instead of forcing change in others, model the behaviors you wish to see and create an environment that encourages personal development. Let people come to their own conclusions.

---

### RELATED PROBLEMS & OBJECTIVES TO REACH:

- **Problem**: Rigid expectations in friendships and relationships can lead to dissatisfaction and unnecessary conflict.

    - **Objective**: Embrace flexibility and non-attachment in relationships, allowing connections to evolve naturally.

- **Problem**: Attempts to pressure others to change often backfire, causing resistance and strain.

    - **Objective**: Use the **ABC Loop** to guide others toward change without exerting pressure, and model the behaviors you wish to see in them.

- **Problem**: Misunderstanding of adult friendship dynamics can lead to feelings of isolation or rejection.

    - **Objective**: Recognize the complexity of adult friendships and be patient as these relationships take time to develop.

---

### ACTION PLAN:

1. **Reflect on Relationship Expectations**: Review your current friendships and relationships. Are you holding onto expectations that might be creating tension or disappointment? Consider letting go of these rigid ideas.

2. **Practice the ABC Loop**: In your next attempt to encourage change in others, apply the **ABC Loop**—start by asking open-ended questions, step back and allow space for growth, and celebrate any progress.

3. **Model Desired Behaviors**: Instead of pushing others to change, focus on embodying the qualities and behaviors you want to see. Create an environment where change can happen naturally.

4. **Be Patient with Relationships**: Understand that adult friendships, especially in the context of life transitions, take time to grow. Invest in casual connections and allow them to evolve organically.

By applying Robbins' framework, you can better navigate adult friendships, foster change in a supportive, non-pressuring way, and reclaim your personal agency in all aspects of life.

In Chapter 16, Robbins delves into the critical distinction between offering support and enabling destructive behaviors. She argues that rescuing individuals from their struggles—whether by shielding them from consequences or solving their problems—ultimately hinders their personal growth and recovery.

Robbins draws on expert insights, particularly from **Dr. Robert Waldinger**, a psychiatrist at Harvard Medical School, who emphasizes the importance of allowing individuals to experience the natural consequences of their actions in order to foster growth. **Dr. Luana Marques**, a clinical psychologist, explains that avoidance—facing challenges indirectly—often deepens underlying issues, rather than solving them.

The chapter highlights Robbins' personal experience with her daughter's anxiety. Initially, Robbins' enabling response—letting her daughter sleep in her room to avoid confronting fears—only reinforced her daughter's avoidance behavior. It wasn't until professional intervention encouraged her daughter to confront her anxiety that real progress occurred.

The chapter discusses the neurological aspects of recovery, noting that the brain's development impacts how support should be tailored for younger individuals versus older ones. Robbins outlines a framework for supporting people through difficult situations: **validating feelings** while maintaining **boundaries, separating one's emotions** from those of the person struggling, and offering comfort while fostering **independence**. The chapter concludes by emphasizing that true improvement often comes from discomfort, such as the pain of addiction reaching a point where the need for sobriety outweighs the fear of confronting the problem.

### KEY INSIGHTS AND TAKEAWAYS:

1. **The Danger of Enabling**: Offering too much help or shielding others from the consequences of their actions prevents growth and recovery.

2. **Allowing Natural Consequences**: People often need to experience the natural results of their choices in order to develop and learn from their mistakes.

3. **Avoidance Deepens Problems**: Avoidance can temporarily reduce stress but ultimately worsens underlying issues, as seen in Robbins' experience with her daughter's anxiety.

4. **Effective Support Requires Boundaries**: While emotional support is crucial, it's equally important to set boundaries to encourage independence and prevent enabling.

5. **The Role of Discomfort in Growth**: Growth often requires facing discomfort directly, as people typically won't change unless the pain of staying the same surpasses the difficulty of confronting their issues.

## PRACTICAL APPLICATION AND ACTION PLAN:

1. **Assess Your Support Strategies**: Reflect on your relationships. Are you enabling behaviors by shielding others from consequences? Consider shifting from rescuing to empowering individuals to face their challenges.

2. **Set Healthy Boundaries**: When supporting others, validate their feelings but also maintain clear boundaries to encourage their independence. Be sure you're offering comfort without taking on their emotional burden.

3. **Encourage Confrontation of Challenges**: Instead of avoiding difficult situations, gently guide others to confront and engage with their issues directly. Let them experience the discomfort of doing so, knowing it will lead to personal growth.

4. **Support Independence, Not Dependence**: Focus on fostering independence by offering support that builds resilience rather than dependency.

### OBJECTIVE & GOALS:

- **Objective**: Shift from enabling behaviors to empowering individuals to take responsibility for their own growth.

- **Goal**: Encourage others to face their fears or issues directly, without providing escape routes or shielding them from the consequences.

### ACTION CHECKLIST:

1. Reflect on situations where you might be enabling behaviors in others.

2. Offer emotional support while encouraging others to take responsibility for their actions.

3. Practice maintaining boundaries that allow for growth and independence.

4.  Be patient with others as they navigate discomfort, knowing that true growth often comes through facing challenges head-on.

By embracing these insights and action plans, you can shift your approach to supporting others in a way that fosters long-term growth and resilience, without reinforcing unhealthy patterns.

## PART 3, CHAPTER 17 SUMMARY: "HOW TO PROVIDE SUPPORT THE RIGHT WAY"

In Chapter 17, Robbins delves into the sensitive topic of providing financial support to struggling adults, particularly within parent-adult child relationships. She stresses that offering financial assistance without clear, enforceable conditions often enables destructive behavior, rather than fostering recovery and growth. Robbins draws a sharp distinction between offering **unconditional love** and **unconditional financial support**, arguing that the latter can inadvertently perpetuate dependency.

Robbins presents two perspectives on hitting "rock bottom"—one from the struggling individual and the other from the support provider. The provider realizes that their financial assistance is prolonging the problem, not solving it. She suggests a **conditional support framework**, where support is tied to measurable goals, such as maintaining sobriety in exchange for housing or achieving academic benchmarks for continued tuition assistance. Importantly, Robbins stresses that these conditions must be consistently enforced, even when it's difficult for both parties involved.

Robbins illustrates this principle through her husband Chris's experience during a business crisis. When his brother refused to help him financially, Chris was forced to confront his failing business and his own alcohol misuse. While initially painful, the lack of financial support prompted necessary personal change and transformation.

The chapter concludes by exploring alternative, non-financial forms of support. Robbins shares her experience with postpartum depression, where her support network provided practical assistance without fostering dependency. She emphasizes that creating environments conducive to healing—while allowing individuals to face the natural consequences of their actions—promotes long-term independence and personal growth better than financial assistance ever could.

### KEY INSIGHTS AND TAKEAWAYS:

1.  **Conditional Financial Support**: Providing financial support without clear boundaries can perpetuate unhealthy behaviors. Conditions, such as sobriety or academic performance, should be tied to continued support to encourage personal growth and responsibility.

2. **Rock Bottom**: The concept of "rock bottom" applies not only to those struggling but also to those offering support. Sometimes, stepping back and allowing someone to face the consequences of their actions leads to real change.

3. **Healthy Support Framework**: Effective support requires clear conditions and consistent enforcement. This may mean letting loved ones struggle and confront their problems in order to grow.

4. **Non-Financial Support**: Providing practical, non-financial assistance—such as emotional support or facilitating recovery through action—helps individuals grow without creating dependency.

## *PRACTICAL APPLICATION AND ACTION PLAN:*

1. **Define Boundaries for Financial Support**: If you're considering financial support for someone, create clear conditions tied to measurable progress (e.g., maintaining sobriety, job-search milestones, academic achievements).

2. **Avoid Enabling**: Reflect on whether your support is enabling the other person's behavior. Consider withdrawing assistance if you realize it's preventing the individual from addressing their issues.

3. **Focus on Non-Financial Support**: Instead of offering money, provide other forms of support—emotional encouragement, helping to find resources, or offering a safe space to work through challenges.

4. **Be Consistent with Boundaries**: Enforce conditions for support consistently, even when it feels difficult. This ensures you are truly helping the person grow rather than merely relieving temporary discomfort.

---

*OBJECTIVE & GOALS:*

- **Objective**: Shift from unconditional financial support to conditional, results-based support that promotes responsibility and growth.

- **Goal**: Encourage independence and recovery by providing support in ways that allow individuals to face consequences and grow from their struggles.

*ACTION CHECKLIST:*

1. Review any ongoing financial support you may be providing to others. Are there clear conditions attached to it?

2. Reflect on whether you're enabling unhealthy behaviors by shielding others from the natural consequences of their actions.

3.  Create a strategy for non-financial support, such as providing emotional encouragement, helping with practical solutions, or connecting individuals with resources.

4.  Set clear boundaries for when and how you will provide financial help, ensuring those boundaries are respected.

By applying these insights and action steps, you can provide more effective and empowering support, allowing others to face challenges and grow while maintaining your own emotional and financial well-being.

## PART 3, CHAPTER 18 SUMMARY: "LET THEM SHOW YOU WHO THEY ARE"

In Chapter 18, Robbins applies her core principles to romantic relationships, focusing on how individuals choose whom and how they love. She argues that people's actions, not their words, truly reveal their feelings, and that an intense desire for connection can often lead individuals to overlook red flags and compromise their standards in potential partners.

Robbins critiques modern dating culture, particularly how digital platforms have transformed romance into a competitive game, often encouraging manipulation and playing hard-to-get. She advocates for authenticity in romantic relationships, stressing that meaningful connections are based on genuine interactions, not strategies. Robbins identifies signs that someone might be "chasing love" rather than choosing it mindfully, such as dismissing problematic behavior or creating unrealistic narratives about the relationship's potential.

The chapter provides a practical framework for evaluating romantic situations. Robbins suggests that individuals should approach their dating experiences as though they were advising a close friend, using a binary lens: either someone makes you a priority, or they do not. She highlights that resistance to defining a relationship often indicates a lack of true commitment. Ultimately, Robbins concludes that finding fulfilling love requires the courage to stay authentic and the wisdom to recognize when a potential partner's actions show that they cannot or will not provide the commitment needed.

### KEY INSIGHTS AND TAKEAWAYS:

1.  **Actions Speak Louder Than Words**: In relationships, people's behaviors reveal their true feelings, not what they say. Pay attention to how a partner acts, not just how they speak.

2. **Chasing Love vs. Choosing Love**: Overemphasizing the desire for connection can cause people to ignore red flags and settle for unhealthy relationships. Mindful love involves setting standards and evaluating potential partners based on their actions.

3. **Avoid Manipulation and Games**: Modern dating often encourages playing games, but authenticity should be the foundation of any meaningful connection. Focusing on honesty rather than manipulation leads to deeper, more fulfilling relationships.

4. **Clarity and Commitment**: Undefined relationships often signal a lack of commitment. If someone truly values you, they will prioritize clear communication and mutual goals.

## PRACTICAL APPLICATION AND ACTION PLAN:

1. **Examine Actions, Not Words**: Reflect on your past or current relationships and consider whether the person's actions align with their words. Are they demonstrating the level of commitment they claim?

2. **Set Clear Standards**: Avoid ignoring red flags or dismissing problematic behavior in the pursuit of connection. Establish and maintain personal standards for what you need in a relationship.

3. **Authenticity in Dating**: When dating, prioritize being genuine over playing games or adhering to social dating norms. Practice transparency and honesty to build authentic connections.

4. **Evaluate Relationship Commitment**: If you're in a relationship (or dating someone), consider whether there's clarity in your connection. Is it defined, or are there vague expectations and uncertainty? If there's resistance to defining the relationship, it may be a sign of a lack of genuine commitment.

---

*OBJECTIVE & GOALS:*

- **Objective**: Establish a clear understanding of the behaviors and standards that are essential for meaningful romantic relationships.

- **Goal**: Cultivate healthy, authentic connections by prioritizing actions over words, recognizing red flags early, and encouraging clear communication and commitment.

---

*ACTION CHECKLIST:*

1. Reflect on past romantic relationships—did you tend to overlook red flags or dismiss behaviors that didn't align with your standards?

2. Make a list of your relationship deal-breakers and non-negotiables. What do you need from a partner to feel valued and respected?

3. Practice being authentic in your dating life. Avoid manipulating situations or falling into competitive dating games.

4. Set boundaries around undefined relationships and insist on clear communication about mutual intentions and goals.

By embracing authenticity and recognizing the signs of true commitment, you can navigate romantic relationships with clarity and confidence, ultimately finding love that aligns with your values and needs.

## PART 3, CHAPTER 19 SUMMARY: "HOW TO TAKE YOUR RELATIONSHIP TO THE NEXT LEVEL"

In Chapter 19, Robbins delves into the challenges individuals face when it comes to relationship commitment. She explores two main scenarios: the chronic pursuit of unavailable partners and the difficulty in advancing an existing relationship.

For those who repeatedly find themselves pursuing unavailable partners, Robbins references research from the University of Alberta, which suggests that these patterns often stem from subconscious influences rooted in childhood and past relationships. She advises individuals in this situation to take a break from dating for at least a year and focus on therapy to help break these ingrained patterns.

For those struggling to progress in a specific relationship, Robbins shares insights from relationship expert Matthew Hussey. Drawing from his own experience with his wife, Audrey, Hussey recommends having in-person conversations focused on personal values and the time investment each partner is willing to make. This approach, based on clarity and alignment of commitment, helped Hussey and Audrey solidify their relationship, ultimately leading to marriage and a business partnership.

Robbins concludes the chapter by addressing the potential negative consequences of commitment discussions. She emphasizes the importance of not maintaining relationships with incompatible commitment levels, framing breakups as necessary steps for finding a more suitable partner in the future.

### KEY INSIGHTS AND TAKEAWAYS:

1. **Breaking Repetitive Relationship Patterns**: Subconscious patterns from past experiences can lead to chronic pursuit of unavailable partners. Taking time to be single and engage in therapy can help break these unhealthy cycles.

2. **Effective Commitment Conversations**: When struggling to advance a relationship, focus on having clear, in-person discussions about your personal values and the level of commitment each partner is willing to invest. Avoid relying solely on emotional appeals.

3. **Recognizing Incompatibility**: If there's a mismatch in commitment levels, it's important to recognize when a relationship isn't serving both partners and to be willing to end it to make room for a more suitable connection.

## PRACTICAL APPLICATION AND ACTION PLAN:

1. **Reflect on Past Relationship Patterns**: If you've experienced repeated patterns of pursuing unavailable partners, consider taking a break from dating and seek therapy to work through the underlying reasons for these behaviors.

2. **Initiate Commitment Conversations**: If you're in a relationship and feel it's not progressing, have an open, honest conversation about your personal values and commitment levels. Prioritize clarity and understanding rather than relying on emotional pleas.

3. **Evaluate Compatibility**: Assess whether your current relationship aligns with your long-term goals. If commitment levels don't match, consider whether it's time to move on and make room for a more compatible partnership.

### OBJECTIVE & GOALS:

- **Objective**: Identify and break negative relationship patterns while fostering healthy, clear commitment conversations to move relationships forward.

- **Goal**: Create a foundation for mutual commitment and clarity in your relationship, leading to long-term compatibility and growth.

### ACTION CHECKLIST:

1. Reflect on any patterns in your past relationships—do you often pursue unavailable partners? Consider taking a break from dating to focus on healing and self-awareness.

2. If you're in a relationship that's not progressing, initiate a conversation about commitment. Focus on clear communication about values and the level of investment each person is willing to make.

3. Assess your relationship's compatibility and make sure both partners are aligned in their long-term goals. If there's misalignment, be open to ending the relationship and seeking a more suitable match.

By addressing and resolving relationship commitment issues with honesty, self-awareness, and clarity, you can pave the way for stronger, healthier connections in your romantic life.

## PART 3, CHAPTER 20 SUMMARY: "HOW EVERY ENDING IS A BEAUTIFUL BEGINNING"

In Chapter 20, Robbins discusses the power of ending relationships and how it can lead to beautiful new beginnings. She highlights two crucial requirements for successful romantic relationships: mutual commitment to improvement and an absence of conflicts that demand abandoning one's core values. Referring to research by John and Julie Gottman, Robbins explains that 69% of relationship problems stem from irreconcilable personality differences or conflicting life goals.

Robbins introduces her ABC approach for managing relationship conflicts: **Apologize and ask questions, Back off and observe behavior**, and **Celebrate progress while modeling desired changes**. She suggests allowing three to six months for change to occur naturally, without pressure.

For relationships that end, Robbins offers strategies for post-breakup recovery, grounded in both scientific research and personal experience. She explains the neurological impact of breakups, noting that romantic relationships become deeply integrated into the nervous system, making separation emotionally difficult. To help with recovery, Robbins outlines six strategies: removing physical reminders, redecorating living spaces, maintaining social connections, scheduling activities, pursuing personal growth, and maintaining hope for future relationships.

The chapter concludes with a shift towards self-love as the foundation of all relationships. Robbins reframes the Let Them Theory as a tool for personal empowerment, focusing on authenticity and self-expression. She emphasizes that by accepting others for who they are, individuals can create space for personal growth and deeper self-understanding.

## CONCLUSION SUMMARY: "YOUR LET ME ERA IS HERE"

In the conclusion, Robbins synthesizes her core message about personal empowerment using the metaphor of weather and sky. Just as we cannot control the weather or others' behaviors, we have complete authority over our responses to external circumstances.

Robbins critiques the mindset that attributes personal limitations to external factors—such as the wealth or success of others—and encourages readers to focus on their own goals and development. She asserts that successful individuals are distinguished by their ability to stay focused on their objectives despite outside pressures. Mental energy spent on worrying about others' opinions or actions only depletes resources that could be better used for personal growth.

The chapter reiterates the two key principles: **Let Them** (allowing others to behave as they choose) and **Let Me** (proactively developing oneself through actionable steps).

Robbins concludes by urging readers to take responsibility for their happiness, energy, and progress, offering a call to action to redirect focus from external factors to personal agency. She assures readers that embracing these principles will lead to positive change, though it requires sustained effort.

## KEY INSIGHTS AND TAKEAWAYS:

1. **The Power of Ending Relationships**: Endings can be painful but are often the catalysts for new beginnings, leading to personal growth and transformation.

2. **Understanding Relationship Dynamics**: Recognize that some relationship issues stem from irreconcilable differences. Understanding this helps you approach relationships with more clarity and less attachment to unrealistic outcomes.

3. **Managing Breakups**: Post-breakup recovery requires practical strategies such as removing reminders, maintaining social connections, and focusing on personal growth to foster healing.

4. **Self-Love as the Foundation of Relationships**: The ultimate foundation for all relationships is self-love. Accepting others as they are, while also embracing personal authenticity, is key to building fulfilling connections.

5. **Empowerment through Personal Agency**: You have control over your responses and actions. Let go of the need to control others and focus on self-development to achieve happiness and progress.

## PRACTICAL APPLICATION AND ACTION PLAN:

1. **Reframe Breakups as Opportunities**: If a relationship ends, view it as a chance for personal growth rather than a loss. Implement the recovery strategies Robbins suggests, focusing on healing and self-improvement.

2. **Use the ABC Approach for Conflict Resolution**: In any current or future relationships, apply the ABC approach (Apologize, Back off, Celebrate) to address issues constructively, allowing time for change without forcing it.

3. **Practice Self-Love and Acceptance**: Prioritize your own well-being and self-growth, knowing that this is the foundation for all other relationships in your life.

4. **Redirect Focus to Personal Goals**: Instead of focusing on external pressures or others' behaviors, channel your energy into your own personal and professional growth. Use the "Let Me" mindset to make actionable progress in your life.

- **Objective**: Embrace the idea that every relationship ending opens up the potential for new beginnings and personal growth.

- **Goal**: Focus on self-love and empowerment, allowing space for authentic self-expression and development in all relationships.

*ACTION CHECKLIST:*

1. Reflect on any past relationship endings and how you've grown from them. Commit to seeing future endings as opportunities for growth.

2. In relationships, apply the ABC approach to manage conflicts constructively and allow time for change.

3. Focus on self-love and self-empowerment. Take actionable steps every day toward personal growth and authenticity.

4. Redirect energy away from external factors and focus on your personal goals, embracing the "Let Me" principle to take control of your progress and happiness.

By implementing these principles, you can create a life where you embrace change, foster healthy relationships, and pursue personal fulfillment with clarity and purpose.

# ANALYSIS OF PART 3, CHAPTER 16-CONCLUSION OF THE LET THEM THEORY

The concluding section of *The Let Them Theory* reinforces the book's key themes of personal agency, non-attachment, and empowering choices in relationships. Through a mix of behavioral psychology, neuroscience, expert research, and personal anecdotes, Robbins offers a powerful framework for navigating challenging interpersonal dynamics, such as supporting loved ones through their struggles and fostering healthy romantic connections.

## KEY THEMES AND CONCEPTS:

1. **Recognizing and Reclaiming Personal Agency:** A central theme in this section is the recognition that individuals often lose their personal power by attempting to control or "rescue" others. Robbins stresses that change must come from within the individual experiencing the challenge—whether it's addiction, mental health, or personal growth. She argues that the desire to "fix" someone else can often be counterproductive, as it enables destructive behaviors instead of fostering independence. The pivotal quote, "You can't want somebody's sobriety or their healing or their financial freedom or their ambition or their happiness more than they do," encapsulates this idea. This principle applies to various contexts, from parenting to romantic relationships, emphasizing that personal transformation is a choice and cannot be imposed by external forces.

2. **Freedom Through Non-Attachment:** Robbins explores how attachment to specific outcomes or behaviors in others, especially in romantic relationships, creates unnecessary suffering. She presents the metaphor of the sky and weather—something uncontrollable, yet navigable. Just as the sky will do what it does, others will behave as they will, and acceptance of this fact offers freedom. The idea is that by letting go of the need to control or fix others, individuals can foster more authentic and fulfilling connections. This theme of freedom through acceptance is essential to the book's message, illustrating how non-attachment can lead to more meaningful relationships.

3. **Redirecting Energy Toward Empowering Choices:** The text emphasizes the importance of consciously redirecting one's energy toward empowering choices—whether through setting boundaries, pursuing personal growth, or making decisions based on internal motivations. Robbins outlines the shift from trying to change others to focusing on what one can control: their actions, responses, and choices. This redirection is crucial for personal development and creates positive change not just in oneself, but also in relationships. Robbins

stresses that this is not an easy process but requires consistent practice, particularly when dealing with loved ones who may not be ready for change.

## RHETORICAL APPROACHES:

Robbins uses a layered approach to convey her message, combining scientific research, case studies, personal anecdotes, and expert testimony to provide a comprehensive understanding of relationship dynamics. This multi-dimensional method creates a balance between theory and practical application. The theoretical frameworks presented early in each chapter are followed by tangible examples that demonstrate the implementation of these principles in real-life situations.

Repetition of key concepts and phrases reinforces the central ideas throughout the book. For instance, Robbins consistently returns to the ideas of "Let Them" (allowing others to be who they are) and "Let Me" (empowering oneself to make choices). These repeated ideas ensure the reader grasps the core principles while maintaining a focus on actionable steps.

### Integration of Psychological and Neuroscientific Research:

The conclusion brings together a variety of psychological and neuroscientific insights, referencing experts like Dr. Robert Waldinger and the Gottmans, to ground Robbins's arguments in research. Studies on addiction, mental health, and attachment patterns strengthen the text's credibility, showing how these theoretical concepts are supported by evidence from behavioral psychology. By referencing established research, Robbins enhances the book's reliability, presenting its arguments as scientifically validated while keeping the language accessible for a broad audience.

### The Sky Metaphor:

The extended metaphor of the sky plays a central role in the book's conclusion, encapsulating the idea that we cannot control external circumstances—like the weather or other people's actions—but we have the power to navigate through them. This metaphor extends beyond relationship dynamics, influencing how individuals approach life's challenges. It serves as a reminder that acceptance of the uncontrollable is essential for personal empowerment, enabling individuals to focus on what they can change: their responses and actions.

### Language and Style:

Robbins's use of clear, relatable language makes complex psychological concepts accessible to a wide audience. The narrative is structured to guide the reader from theoretical understanding to practical application, ensuring that the principles are not only understood but can be integrated into everyday life. Direct address and the use of rhetorical devices like repetition and metaphor ensure the book remains engaging and encourages readers to reflect on how they can apply these concepts to their own lives.

## CONCLUSION:

The final chapters of *The Let Them Theory* provide a thoughtful and practical framework for navigating relationships and personal growth. By emphasizing personal agency, non-attachment, and the redirection of energy toward empowering choices, Robbins offers a roadmap for cultivating healthy relationships and fostering self-improvement. The integration of scientific research, expert testimony, and personal anecdotes strengthens the text's credibility and applicability. Ultimately, the conclusion ties together the book's themes, urging readers to take control of their own happiness and responses to external challenges, while allowing others the freedom to make their own choices. Through this, Robbins empowers her audience to embrace life's unpredictability and create meaningful, authentic connections.

Manufactured by Amazon.ca
Acheson, AB